DASH Diet

SMOOTHIES
Delicious and Nutritious Smoothies for Great Health

Robertina Whelans

Ordinary Matters Publishing

DASH DIET SMOOTHIES
Delicious and Nutritious Smoothies for Great Health
Ordinary Matters Publishing
Ordinary MattersPublishing.com

DISCLAIMER: The recipes within this book, DASH DIET SMOOTH-IES, are for information purposes only and are not meant as a diet to treat, prescribe, or diagnose illness. Please seek the advice of a doctor or alternative health care professional if you have any health issues you would like addressed or before you begin any diet.

Book Layout © 2014 BookDesignTemplates.com

DASH DIET SMOOTHIES / Robertina Whelans-1st Ed.
ASIN: B00J2GXKN2 (eBook)
ISBN-10: 1941303129 (print)
ISBN-13: 978-1-941303-12-2 (print)

https://www.amazon.com/author/dashdiet

www.facebook.com/DASH-Diet-Smoothies-and-Recipes

"Your diet is a bank account.
Good food choices are good investments."

—BETHANY FRANKEL

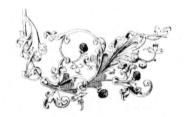

CONTENTS

INTRODUCTION

With an estimated seven out of ten Americans now taking at least one prescription drug, the emphasis on achieving good health is now stronger than it has ever been.

Ranked as one of the healthiest diets, and the best diet for diabetes four years in a row, the DASH diet has been hailed as "the diet for all diseases," and has been proven to improve health over a variety of conditions.

The DASH diet stands for Dietary Approaches to Stop Hypertension. It was originally developed by the US National Institute of Health, as a way to lower blood pressure without medication.

By following the dietary advice within the DASH diet, it is possible to reduce your blood pressure by a few points in as little as two weeks. Prolonged use of the diet can see systolic blood pressure reduced by as much as 12 points, which is significant in treating high blood pressure and its resultant effects.

Lowered risk of heart disease, stroke, cholesterol, kidney failure, and several types of cancer, are all benefits of the DASH diet. More so, with its emphasis on real foods, especially fruits and vegetables, and the right amount of protein, the DASH diet has proven itself to be a great weight loss tool.

However, incorporating the principles of the DASH diet should be a lifestyle practice and not just a short term solution to health problems or weight loss.

Our intention with this book is to show you how easy it is to make the changes necessary to change your diet. Starting with fruits and vegetables, we will show you how simple it is to increase your daily intake, through delicious and nutritious smoothies.

Guidelines of the DASH Diet

The DASH Diet is an eating plan that is high in potassium, magnesium, and calcium. It is low in sodium, rich in fruits and vegetables, and low in fat or non-fat dairy.

Grains, especially whole grains, lean meat, fish, poultry, and nuts and beans make up the rest of the diet. High in fiber and low in fat, it is a healthier way of eating, flexible enough to adapt to the lifestyles of most people.

For the purposes of this book, we are going to concentrate on the fruit and vegetable part of the diet. An abundance of fruits and vegetables can be eaten with the DASH diet.

The following are the guidelines to aim for:

Vegetables — 4 to 5 servings per day
1 serving equals:
1 cup raw leafy vegetables
1/2 cup of cut—up raw or cooked vegetables
1/2 cup vegetable juice
Fruit — 4 to 5 servings per day
1 serving equals:
1 medium fruit
1/4 cup dried fruit
1/2 cup fresh, frozen or canned fruit
1/2 cup fruit juice

You are also allowed low fat (or fat free) milk products with this diet, which can be used success-fully in smoothies.

Milk — 2 to 3 servings per day
1 serving equals:
1 cup of milk or yogurt

Additional Notes

ABOUT SMOOTHIES

What Are Smoothies?

Smoothies are blended drinks made predominately from fruits. However, they can also be made from leafy green vegetables. While the diet calls usually calls for low fat milk and/or dairy products, many people add soy or almond milk, nut milks, various nut butters and even dairy—free yogurts to their smoothies.

> *Milk substitutes such as soy, or rice milk / yogurt / cheeses can also be used, just make sure these substitutes have the same amount of calcium and vitamin D as the original foods.* —*The DASH DIET EATING PLAN*

What Are Their Benefits?

You'll find many health benefits to drinking smoothies and you can expect to experience at least some of these:

Improved hydration – smoothies are full of water, from the fruits and veggies to the dairy products, which are largely water. Drinking a smoothie for breakfast is a good way to ensure that you start the day fully hydrated.

Increased energy, focus and mental clarity – increasing your intake for fruits and vegetables will leave you with bags of energy. In turn, this will lead to increased focus and mental clarity. No more brain fog!

Better sleep – a body that is well hydrated and full of the right nutrition, functions in a better way. This includes sleep.

Release of toxins – giving the body good nutrition, in an easily assimilable form, such as liquids, allows it time to "clean house" and release toxins that have built up over time.

Improved digestion and bowel movements – eating a natural diet that is full of fruits, vegetables and fiber, means that our digestive systems work better, and our bowel movements become more regular.

Better immune system – eating a diet that is full of essential nutrients, vitamins and anti—oxidants, ensures our immune systems are working to the best of their ability. You can expect less colds, bugs and infections when eating this way.

Why Are DASH Smoothies Good for You?

Many smoothies on the market today are made from fruit concentrates, syrups and added sugars, preservatives and flavorings.

DASH smoothies follow the dietary principles laid out by the DASH diet. No sugar-filled concentrates, syrups, or preservatives. Clean eating is emphasized. Fresh is definitely best, and with a DASH smoothie you are guaranteed goodness with none of those nasty ingredients.

What Equipment Do You Need?

All you need to make smoothies is a blender or a smoothie maker. If you use a blender, make sure it has a 2—3 liter jug on it. Note: the higher the speed of your blender, the easier it will be to completely blend your smoothies.

How to Get Started

Simply make sure you have a good variety of fruits, low-fat milk, soy or almond milk substitutes — and leafy green vegetables on hand. Best to buy organic produce where possible. A good starting point would be to have:

At least 6 oranges
Spinach or kale
A selection of fruits and berries

Low fat milk or soy, plant-based, or almond
Low fat or dairy-free yogurt

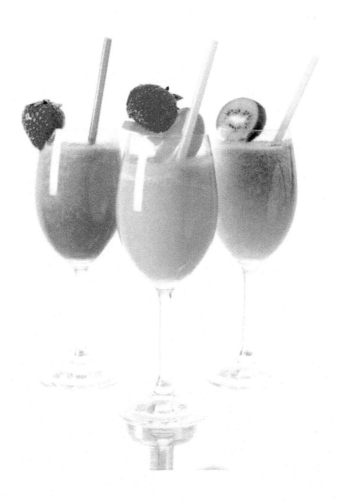

SMOOTHIE RECIPES

The following recipes offer a wide variety of breakfast, lunch, dinner, and dessert recipes. Nutritional information is provided at the end of each recipe. Remember:

> *Milk substitutes such as soy, or rice milk / yogurt / cheeses can also be used, just make sure these substitutes have the same amount of calcium and vitamin D as the original foods. —The DASH DIET EATING PLAN*

NOTE: Most recipes make one large smoothie or can be divided into two.

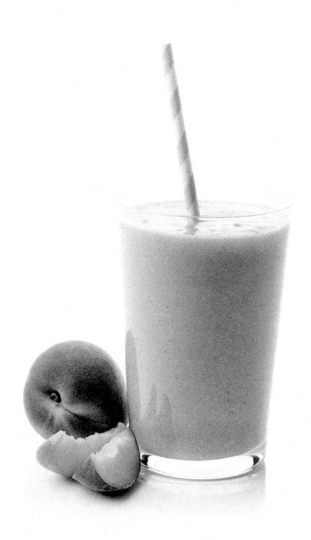

ORANGE SMOOTHIES

Freshly squeezed orange juice makes a perfect base for smoothie recipes. Orange juice is a great source of vitamin C. An essential vitamin that cannot be synthesized by the body, it protects against the signs of early aging and tissue damage.

Orange Peach Smoothie

Servings: 1 to 2

Ingredients:
2 cups freshly squeezed orange juice (1 large or 2 small oranges)
1 peach, de-stoned and cut into slices
1 mango, peeled and cut into slices

Instructions:
Combine the ingredients in a high-speed blender.

Blend the mixture on high speed for 30 to 60 seconds until thoroughly combined and smooth.

Add water for a thinner consistency.

Pour the smoothie into glasses and enjoy immediately.

Nutritional Information:
426 calories per serving, 2g fat, 103g carbs, 6g protein, 7g fiber, 9.1 sodium

Strawberry-Orange Ice

Servings: 1 to 2

Ingredients:
1 cup frozen squeezed orange juice
7 large or 14 small strawberries

Instructions:
Combine the ingredients in a high-speed blender.

Blend the mixture on high speed for 30 to 60 seconds until thoroughly combined.

Pour the smoothie into glasses and enjoy immediately.

Nutritional Information:
491.9 calories per serving, .98g fat, 118g carbs, 7.63g protein, 4.79g fiber, 9.78 sodium

Orange and Apricot Smoothie

Servings: 1 to 2

Ingredients:
1 cup freshly squeezed orange juice
1/2 cup canned apricots in fruit juice; no sugar
1 cup white seedless grapes

Instructions:
Drain apricots.

Add all ingredients in a blender.

Blend until smooth.

Pour the smoothie into glasses and enjoy immediately.

Nutritional Information:
200 calories per serving, 0g fat, 50g carbs, 2g protein, 5g fiber

Tangerine and Papaya Delight

Servings: 1 to 2

Ingredients:
2 tangerines
1 cup papaya, peeled and sliced
1 cup freshly squeezed tangerine juice or water

Instructions:
Add all the ingredients.

Blend until smooth.

Pour the smoothie into glasses and enjoy immediately.

Nutritional Information:
160 calories per serving, 3g fat, 32g carbs, 3g protein, 5g fiber

Orange Twister Smoothie

Servings: 1 to 2

Ingredients
1 cup freshly squeezed orange juice
1 banana, cut into one inch chunks
1/2 lime, peeled
1/2 cup crushed ice.

Instructions:
Combine the ingredients in a blender.

Blend the mixture until thoroughly combined.

Pour the smoothie into glasses and enjoy immediately.

Nutritional Information:
280 calories per serving, 9.5g fat, 22g carbs, 6.5g protein, 14g fiber

---

Additional Notes

Use this section to make additional notes.

_____

_____

_____

_____

_____

_____

_____

_____

_____

_____

_____

_____

_____

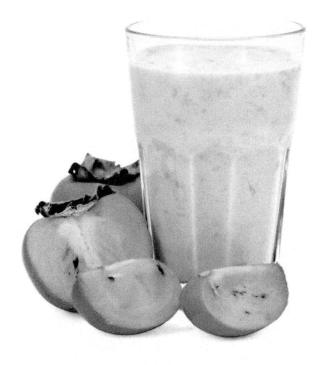

MILK SMOOTHIES

On the DASH diet, you are allowed fat-free milk and associated products. Milk and yogurts work well in smoothies, so here are a few recipes to get your started.

Blackberry Cream Smoothie

Servings: 1 to 2

Ingredients:
1/2 cup fresh blackberries (fresh or frozen)
1/2 banana
1/2 - 1 cup low fat milk or fat-free milk or almond milk

Instructions:
Combine the ingredients in a blender.

Blend the mixture until smooth.

Pour the smoothie into glasses and enjoy immediately.

Nutritional Information:
120 calories per serving, 0g fat, 27.5g carbs, 4g protein, 6g fiber

Strawberry-Cucumber Smoothie

Servings: 1 to 2

Ingredients:
1/2 cup frozen strawberries
1 cup low fat or fat-free or almond milk
1/2 cucumber, chopped or sliced
1/2 tbsp. honey
Squeeze of lemon, optional

Instructions:
Combine the ingredients in blender.

Blend the mixture until thoroughly combined.

Pour the smoothie into glasses.

Nutritional Information:
225 calories per serving, 20g fat, 14g carbs, 3g protein, 8g fiber

---

Chocolate Banana Smoothie

Servings: 1 to 2

Ingredients:
1 banana
1 tsp. good quality unsweetened cocoa powder
1 cup low fat or fat-free milk or almond milk

Instructions:
Combine the ingredients in a blender.

Blend the mixture until thoroughly combined.

Pour the smoothie into glasses and enjoy immediately.

Nutritional Information:
120 calories per serving, 1g fat, 26g carbs, 3g protein, 2.5g fiber

_____

_____

_____

_____

Spicy Mandarin Smoothie

Servings: 1 to 2

Ingredients:

1/2 cup low fat or fat—free or almond milk
1 large, or 2 small mandarins, peeled and seeded.
1 cup frozen mango chunks
1 tbsp. honey
1/8 tsp. cayenne pepper

Instructions:

Combine the ingredients in a blender.

Blend the mixture until thoroughly combined.

Pour the smoothie into glasses and enjoy immediately.

Nutritional Information:

150 calories per serving, 0.5g fat, 38g carbs, 1g protein, 1.5g fiber

Pineapple-Ginger Smoothie

Servings: 1 to 2

Ingredients:
1 cup fresh or frozen pineapple—cut into pieces
1/2 inch fresh ginger
1 cup low fat or fat-free yogurt
1/2 cup low fat or fat—free milk or almond milk
1/8 tsp. ground cinnamon

Instructions:
Combine the ingredients in a blender.

Blend the mixture until thoroughly combined.

Pour the smoothie into glasses and enjoy immediately.

Nutritional Information:
130 calories per serving, 1g fat, 31g carbs, 2g protein, 3g fiber

Additional Notes

Use this section to make additional notes.

_____

_____

_____

_____

_____

_____

_____

_____

_____

_____

_____

_____

_____

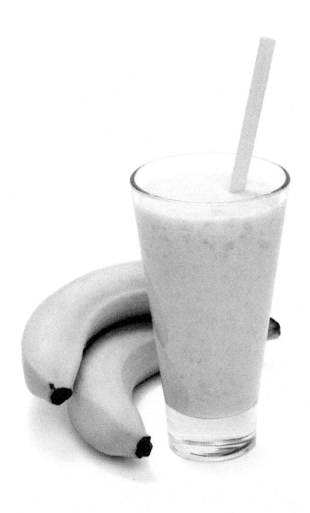

BANANA SMOOTHIES

Bananas are low in sodium and high in potassium, so they are a good addition to your DASH diet. Bananas can be used successfully in most smoothies, so feel free to play around with them. Add them to different recipes to see how the newly made smoothies taste. The following are just a few examples to get you started.

Summer Holiday in a Glass

Servings: 1 to 2

Ingredients:

1 mango, peeled and cut into slices
1 cup pineapple, peeled and into slices
1 cup unsweetened coconut water
1 banana

Instructions:

Combine the ingredients in a blender.

Blend the mixture until thoroughly combined.

Pour the smoothie into glasses and enjoy immediately.

Nutritional Information:

140 calories per serving, 3g fat, 27g carbs, 3g protein, 4g fiber

_____

_____

_____

Banana Date Smoothie

Servings: 1 to 2

Ingredients:

2 bananas, peeled and chopped
1 cup water
3 medjool dates

Instructions:

Combine the ingredients in a blender.

Blend the mixture until thoroughly combined.

Pour the smoothie into glasses and enjoy immediately.

Nutritional Information:

220 calories per serving, 8g fat, 34g carbs, 4g protein, 6g fiber

Banana and Coconut Smoothie

Servings: 1 to 2

Ingredients:

1 large frozen banana
1/2 cup chopped Romaine lettuce
1 cup coconut water
14 chopped medjool date
1/4 tsp. vanilla essence

Instructions:

Combine the ingredients in a blender.

Blend the mixture until thoroughly combined.

Pour the smoothie into glasses and enjoy immediately.

Nutritional Information:

260 calories per serving, 12g fat, 6g carbs, 6.5g protein, 2g fiber

Additional Notes

Use this section to make additional notes.

_____

_____

_____

_____

_____

_____

_____

_____

_____

_____

_____

_____

_____

_____

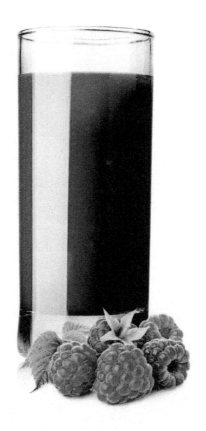

YOGURT SMOOTHIES

Yogurt is a long-time favorite of the health crowd as it has a number of benefits. In addition to being a great source of calcium, vitamins B-2, B-12, as well as potassium and magnesium are found. In recent years the additional benefit of probiotics has made yogurt increase in value.

Orange Cream Smoothie

Servings: 1 to 2

Ingredients:

1 cup freshly squeezed orange juice
1/2 cup low fat or fat-free yogurt
1/2 cup low fat or fat-free or almond milk

Instructions:

Combine the ingredients in a blender.

Blend until smooth and well combined.

Pour the smoothie into glasses and enjoy immediately.

Nutritional Information:

360 calories per serving, 23g fat, 36g carbs, 9g protein, 8g fiber

_____

_____

_____

Mango Juice Smoothie

Servings: 1 to 2

Ingredients:

1 large mango—peeled and diced
1 banana, cut into chunks
1/2 cup low fat or fat-free yogurt
1 cup freshly squeezed orange juice

Instructions:

Combine the ingredients in a blender.

Blend the mixture until thoroughly combined.

Pour the smoothie into glasses and enjoy immediately.

Nutritional Information:

120 calories per serving, 3.5g fat, 14g carbs, 8.5g protein, 2g fiber

_____

_____

_____

Dreamy Raspberry Smoothie

Servings: 1 o 2

Ingredients:

1 cup low fat or fat-free yogurt
1/2 cup low fat or fat-free milk
1 cup frozen raspberries
3/4 cup strawberries

Instructions:

Combine the ingredients in a blender.

Blend the mixture until thoroughly combined.

Pour the smoothie into glasses and enjoy immediately.

Nutritional Information:

220 calories per serving, 8g fat, 33g carbs, 10g protein, 7g fiber

Berry Ulta-Nice Smoothie

Servings: 1 to 2

Ingredients:

1/2 cup pineapple—peeled and chopped
1/2 cup blackberries
1/2 cup blueberries
1/2 cup low fat or fat-free yogurt
1/2 cup low fat or fat-free milk

Instructions:

Combine the ingredients in a blender.

Blend the mixture until thoroughly combined.

Pour the smoothie into glasses and enjoy immediately.

Nutritional Information:

185 calories per serving, 7.5g fat, 23g carbs, 10g protein, 3.5g fiber

Mangolicious Smoothie

Servings: 1 to 2

Ingredients:

1 ripe mango, peeled and chopped
1 banana
1/2 cup pineapple, peeled and sliced
1/2 cup low fat or fat-free yogurt

Instructions:

Combine the ingredients in a blender.

Blend the mixture until thoroughly combined.

Pour the smoothie into glasses and enjoy immediately.

Nutritional Information:

185 calories per serving, 5g fat, 25g carbs, 9g protein, 2g fiber

_____

_____

_____

Additional Notes

Use this section to make additional notes.

_____

_____

_____

_____

_____

_____

_____

_____

_____

_____

_____

_____

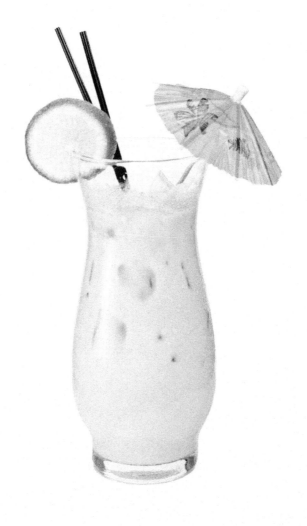

GREEN SMOOTHIES

Green smoothies, made with leafy green vegetables, are rich in magnesium, potassium and calcium, all of which make up an important part of the DASH diet.

Sunshine Smoothie

Servings: 1 to 2

Ingredients:
1 cup spinach
1 cup collard greens or kale
1/2 cup of pineapple, cut in chunks
1 cup of freshly squeezed orange juice

Instructions:
Combine the ingredients in a blender.

Blend the mixture until thoroughly combined.

Pour the smoothie into glasses and enjoy immediately.

Nutritional Information:
265 calories per serving, 0.5g fat, 67g carbs, 2g protein, 6g fiber

_____

_____

_____

Breakfast Smoothie

Servings: 1 to 2

Ingredients:
1 cup of freshly squeezed orange juice
1 mango—peeled and sliced
1 cup spinach
1 banana
Water, if needed

Instructions:
Combine the ingredients in a blender.

Blend the mixture until thoroughly combined.

Pour the smoothie into glasses and enjoy immediately.

Nutritional Information:
180 calories per serving, 4g fat, 38g carbs, 1g protein, 5g fiber

Cilantro Lemonade Smoothie

Servings: 1 to 2

Ingredients:
3/4 cup spinach
1/4 cup cilantro
1 cup water
1 banana, cut into chunks
1/2 lime, peeled
1/2 inch fresh ginger

Instructions:
Rinse the spinach.

Add all ingredients into a blender.

Blend the mixture until thoroughly combined.

Nutritional Information:
155 calories per serving, 0g fat, 35g carbs, 5g protein

Berry-Banana Greens Smoothie

Servings: 1 to 2

Ingredients:
1 cup spinach
1/2 cup water
1/2 cup freshly squeezed orange juice
1/2 cup strawberries
1/2 cup blueberries
1 banana

Instructions:
Combine the ingredients in a blender.

Blend the mixture until thoroughly combined.

Pour the smoothie into glasses and enjoy immediately.

Nutritional Information:
230 calories per serving, 1g fat, 57g carbs, 2g protein, 3g fiber

_____

_____

Peachy Coconut Dream Smoothie

Servings: 1 to 2

Ingredients:
1 cup spinach, freshly rinsed
1 cup coconut water
1 cup white seedless grapes
1 peach—stoned and sliced
5 to 6 drops almond extract

Instructions:
Remove the pit from the peach and slice.

Combine the ingredients in a blender.

Blend the mixture until thoroughly combined.

Pour the smoothie into glasses and enjoy immediately.

Nutritional Information:
185 calories per serving, 8g fat, 25g carbs, 4.5g protein, 1.5g fiber

Additional Notes

Use this section to make additional notes.

_____

_____

_____

_____

_____

_____

_____

_____

_____

_____

_____

_____

_____

_____

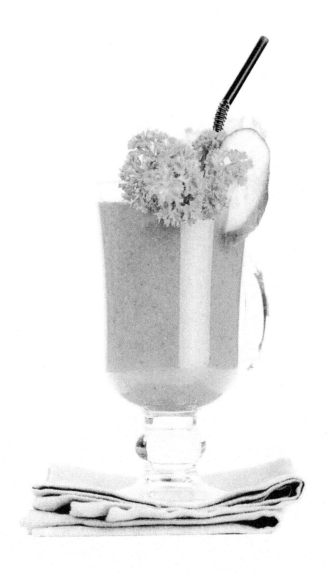

CELERY SMOOTHIES

Celery can be a very useful vegetable in bringing down high blood pressure, so its place in the DASH diet is well deserved. In addition to celery being loaded with vitamins and minerals, this great green is full of beneficial enzymes, as well as antioxidants.

Green Celery Smoothie

Servings: 1 to 2

Ingredients:
1 small banana
2 medium stalks of celery, cut into small chunks
1 cup spinach
1/2 cup water
1/2 cup pineapple—peeled and chopped

Instructions:
Add the ingredients one at a time to a blender, adding a little water when needed to ensure the right consistency.

Blend the mixture until thoroughly combined.

Pour the smoothie into glasses and enjoy.

Nutritional Information:
170 calories per serving, 0.5g fat, 42g carbs, 2.6g protein, 5g fiber

Red Berry Celery Smoothie

Servings: 1 to 2

Ingredients:
2 medium stalks of celery, cut into chunks
1 banana
1 Honeycrisp apple or other red apple
1/2 cup frozen strawberries
1/2 cup frozen raspberries
1/2 cup water

Instructions:
Combine the ingredients in a blender.

Blend the mixture until thoroughly combined.

Pour the smoothie into glasses and enjoy.

Nutritional Information:
240 calories per serving, 1.5g fat, 56g carbs, 4g protein, 4.5g fiber

Apple-Raspberry and Celery Smoothie

Servings: 1 to 2

Ingredients:
1 cup spinach, rinsed
1 green apple, cut in small chunks
2 small stalks of celery, cut into smaller chunks
1/2 cucumber—peeled and sliced
1/2 cup water
1/2 cup frozen raspberries (unsweetened)

Instructions:
Combine the ingredients in a blender.

Blend the mixture until thoroughly combined.

Pour the smoothie into glasses and enjoy.

Nutritional Information:
150 calories per serving, 2g fat, 34g carbs, 3g protein, 6.5g fiber

Celery & Pineapple-Parsley Blast Smoothie

Servings: 1 to 2

Ingredients:
1 small banana, cut into small chunks
1 medium stalk of celery, cut in small chunks
1/2 cup pineapple—peeled and chopped
1/2 cup water
1 cup parsley

Instructions:
Combine the ingredients in a blender.

Blend the mixture until thoroughly combined.

Pour the smoothie into glasses and enjoy.

Nutritional Information:
115 calories per serving, 2g fat, 22g carbs, 1g protein, 4g fiber

Additional Notes
Use this section to make additional notes.

_____

_____

_____

_____

_____

_____

_____

_____

_____

_____

_____

_____

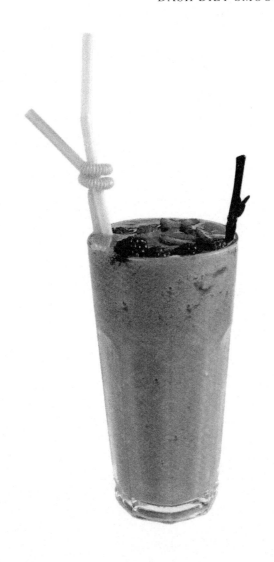

GINGER SMOOTHIES

Ginger contains good amounts of magnesium and potassium, so it is perfect for including in our DASH diet smoothies. Scientific studies continue to promote the many health benefits of ginger, including its strong antioxidant and anti-inflammatory medicinal properties

Orange Ginger Smoothie

Servings: 1 to 2

Ingredients:
1 cup freshly squeezed orange juice
1 large carrot, cut in medium chunks
1/2 cup ginger, sliced
1/4 cup water

Instructions:

Combine the ingredients in a *high-speed* blender. (Because carrots are hard vegetables, you will need the additional power provided by a higher speed.)

Blend all the items except for the carrots.

Then add the carrot pieces, a few at a time, until the mixture has a smooth consistency. Add water as needed.

Pour the smoothie into glasses and enjoy.

Nutritional Information:
291 calories per serving, 3.1g fat, 63.5g carbs, 6.2g protein, 7.7g fiber, 67mg sodium

Apricot Ginger Blast Smoothie

Servings: 1 to 2

Ingredients:

2 fresh apricots, stoned and sliced
1 green apple, de-cored and sliced
1 small stalk of celery
1 cup fresh spinach
1/2 inch fresh ginger
1/2 cup water

Instructions:
Combine the ingredients in a blender.

Blend the mixture until thoroughly combined. (Add more water if needed to get the right consistency.)

Pour the smoothie into glasses and enjoy.

Nutritional Information:
299 calories per serving, 15g fat, 42.1g carbs, 4.5g protein, 7.7g fiber, 784mg sodium

Lemon Ginger Smoothie

Servings: 1 to 2

Instructions:
Juice of one lemon
1 green apple, cut in chunks
1 inch piece of ginger root, quartered
1/2 cup water

Instructions:
Combine the ingredients in a blender.

Blend the mixture until thoroughly combined.

Pour the smoothie into glasses and enjoy.

Nutritional Information:
136 calories per serving, 0.7g fat, 36.3g carbs, 0.9g protein, 5.7g fiber, 7 sodium

_____

_____

_____

_____

_____

Banana Ginger Smoothie

Servings: 1 to 2

Ingredients:
1 banana
3/4 cup low fat or fat-free yogurt
1 tsp. honey
1 1-inch slice of fresh ginger

Instructions:
Combine the ingredients in a blender.

Blend the mixture until thoroughly combined.

Pour the smoothie into glasses and enjoy.

Nutritional Information:
236 calories per serving, 0.8g fat, 48.1g carbs, 12g protein, 3.2g fiber, 144 sodium

_____

_____

_____

Additional Notes

Use this section to make additional notes.

_____

_____

_____

_____

_____

_____

_____

_____

_____

_____

_____

_____

_____

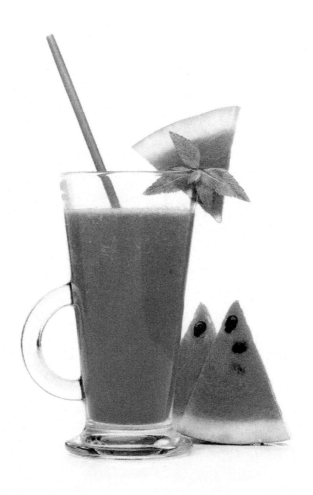

FUN SMOOTHIES

Delicious and fun to whip up, these great smoothie recipes are perfect for a once-a-week treat. Remember, while you're having fun drinking them, they are providing you with plenty of nutrients, fiber, protein, and all sorts of good stuff. As these are true healthy treats, you'll want to drunk them every week—if you're serious about your DASH diet.

Peanut Butter Smoothie

Servings: 1 to 2

Ingredients:
1 banana
1/4 cup peanut butter
1/4 tsp. ground cinnamon
1 cup low fat or fat-free milk or almond milk

Instructions:
Combine the ingredients in a blender.

Blend the mixture until thoroughly combined.

Pour the smoothie into glasses and enjoy.

Nutritional Information:
575 calories per serving, 32.9g fat, 52.1g carbs, 25.4g protein, 7.2g fiber, 428 sodium

---

4th of July Smoothie

Servings: 1 to 2

Ingredients:
1 cup low fat or fat-free milk or almond milk
1 cup frozen strawberries
1 cup frozen blueberries
1/2 cup low fat or fat-free yogurt
1/2 tsp. vanilla extract
1/3 cup unsweetened coconut flakes (reduced fat)
1/2 tsp. honey

Instructions:
Combine the ingredients in a blender.

Blend the mixture until thoroughly combined.

Pour the smoothie into glasses and enjoy.

Nutritional Information:
402 calories per serving, 8.7g fat, 63.9g carbs, 17.5g protein, 9.2g fiber, 226 sodium

Fruity Ice Cream Smoothie

Servings: 1 to 2

Ingredients:
1/2 cup fresh strawberries
1/2 cup fresh raspberries
1/2 cup blueberries
1 medium peach, de-stoned and sliced
1 banana
1 cup low fat or fat-free milk or almond milk
1/2 cup low-fat vanilla ice cream

Instructions:
Combine the ingredients in a blender.

Blend the mixture until thoroughly combined.

Pour the smoothie into glasses and enjoy.

Nutritional Information:
419 calories per serving, 5.2g fat, 84.3g carbs, 13.6g protein, 12.8g fiber, 160 sodium

Chocolate Berry Smoothie

Servings: 1 to 2

Ingredients:
1 tbsp. good quality unsweetened cocoa powder
1 cup frozen raspberries
1 cup frozen strawberries
1 cup low fat or fat-free milk or almond milk

Instructions:
Combine the ingredients in a blender.

Blend the mixture until thoroughly combined.

Pour the smoothie into glasses and enjoy.

Nutritional Information:
410 calories per serving, 0.5g fat, 93.3g carbs, 10.8g protein, 15.8g fiber, 134 sodium

_____

_____

_____

_____

Banana Split Smoothie

Servings: 1 to 2

Ingredients:
1 banana
1 cup pineapple-peeled and cut into pieces
1 cup low fat or fat free milk or almond milk
1/2 cup strawberries
1 scoop low-fat vanilla ice cream

Instructions:
Combine the ingredients in a blender.

Blend the mixture until thoroughly combined.

Pour the smoothie into glasses and enjoy.

Nutritional Information:
0 calories per serving, 0g fat, 0g carbs, 0g protein, 0g fiber, 0 sodium

_____

_____

_____

_____

Additional Notes

Use this section to make additional notes.

_____

_____

_____

_____

_____

_____

_____

_____

_____

_____

_____

_____

CONCLUSION

There is a saying that "health is wealth," and it is a statement that is especially true in a society where one in three people suffer from high blood pressure.

Having high blood pressure can not only cause a risk of heart disease, kidney disease and stroke, but it can also increase the chances of developing certain cancers, diabetes, osteoporosis, and many other diseases.

It makes sense that the more we look after our health, the better our chances of not developing any of these potential life threatening diseases becomes.

The DASH diet offers the perfect solution. A food plan that is easy to follow, interesting to eat, and won't leave you feeling like you are constantly on a "diet." The great indirect effects of following this eating plan will also see you losing weight. It really is a win-win situation.

Taking the time to incorporate the principles of the DASH diet into your lifestyle, on a permanent basis, is certainly a step worth aiming for.

If you think this diet lifestyle might be right for you, this cookbook is the perfect place to begin. Simply choose a recipe from this book and get started. You will not be disappointed. Then grab the other cookbooks in the *DASH Diet Cookbook* series.

Yes, You've Done It!

Congratulations! You've made it to the end of this cookbook. I hope this is only the beginning of an adventure for you into a whole new lifestyle with an emphasis on clean eating and a healthy lifestyle.

Get Your Free copy of DASH Diet Tips, Strategies, and Success Stories now.

GET YOUR FREE DASH DIET BONUS

DASH Diet Tips, Strategies, and Success Stories

Go to: www.MyDashDietCookbooks.com

My DASH Diet Cookbook Series:

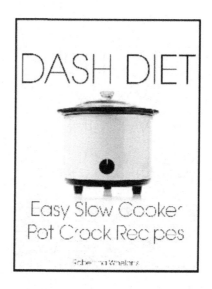

DASH DIET EASY SLOW COOKER
CROCK POT RECIPES

30+ mouthwatering recipes that will save you time. These good clean eating, delicious, quick and easy slow-cooker recipes are gluten-free and dairy-free. You'll find recipes for breakfast, dinner, soups and stews, and dessert recipes, all for one-pot slow cooking.

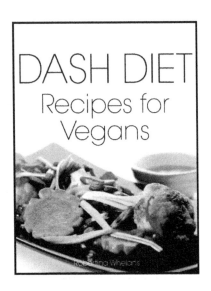

DASH DIET RECIPES for VEGANS

Looking for DASH Diet recipes Vegan-style? While lean meat is allowed on the standard DASH diet, this recipe collection focuses on recipes designed for vegans who wish to give the diet a try. Vegans and vegetarians want to modify the DASH diet, so this collection helps them make that transition. You'll find plenty of tips to help.

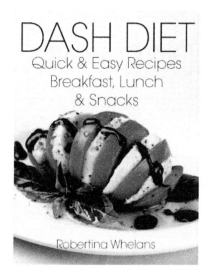

DASH DIET QUICK & EASY RECIPES for BREAKFAST, LUNCH, & SNACKS

Inside this collection, you'll find easy and tasty meals that you can enjoy while on the DASH Diet. No need for guess work. Enjoy recipes for granola bars, panini, wraps, and even pizza bites.

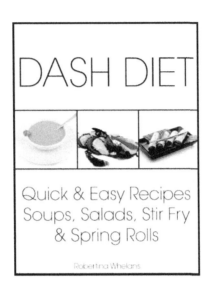

DASH DIET QUICK & EASY RECIPES
SOUPS, SALADS, STIR FRY & SPRING ROLES

Looking for light and easy recipes that incorporate the DASH diet plan? This collection focuses on just that. Inside you'll find recipes like Ginger Veggie Spring Rolls, Asian Veggie Salad with Snow Peas, Shrimp and Tomato Stir-Fry, and even Tuscan White Bean Vegetable Soup and so much more.

About the Author

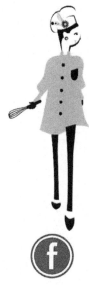

Like my DASH Diet Smoothies and Recipes page.
www.facebook.com/DASH Diet Smoothies and
Recipes

Robertina Whelans first learned of the DASH Diet when she was diagnosed with hypertension and found it to be an effective way to lower her blood pressure. Today, she seeks to share what she's learned about the DASH Diet with others so they, too, can reap similar rewards

Follow my Amazon Author Page
amazon.com/author/RobertinaWhelans

Enjoyed this Cookbook?

I hope you've enjoyed this collection of smoothie recipes and hope you let others know about the DASH Diet, its benefits, and my DASH Diet cookbook series. Like every other author, I do my best to put together a book that my readers will enjoy and find helpful.

One feature you may enjoy more and more as time goes by are the blank lined pages in the paperback editions.

Also, your feedback is crucial to the success of authors like me who are helped by the readers who have read, enjoyed, and found their books useful or helpful, and who are then happy to let others know. If you have enjoyed this book, I'd be grateful if you would take a few minutes to leave an honest review on Amazon or wherever you either bought the book or wherever you enjoy sharing your reading experiences.

Thank you!

Robertina Whelans

NOTES

_____

_____

_____

_____

_____

_____

_____

_____

_____

_____

_____

_____

_____

_____

_____

_____

_____

_____

_____

_____

_____

_____

_____

_____

_____

_____

_____

_____

_____

_____

_____

_____

_____

_____

_____

_____

_____

_____

_____

_____

INDEX

Made in the USA
Columbia, SC
22 April 2020